New Job: Dad

The New Parent Collection, Volume 2

Kelly Mager

Published by Mini Mischief Managed, 2021.

NEW JOB: DAD

First edition. September 16, 2021.

ISBN: 979-8201700751

Written by Kelly Mager.

Table of Contents

For all the moms that made me realize there needed to be a dad's version of "15 Ways For New Moms To Manage Stress & Stay Sane"!

Foreword

Every relationship we have in our lives is constantly changing and shifting as we encounter new experiences. As we learn and grow, our connections to others, and indeed to our own selves, will evolve and grow as well. Major life events can often cause a disruption in even our most stable relationships. However, navigating these events properly can lead to coming through even stronger.

The birth of a child is definitely among one of the most major, life-changing events someone can experience – and it doesn't matter if it's their first child, or their fourth, the dynamic is going to change. Not only will there be a shift in the general family dynamic, but each parent will experience their own changes in responsibilities, expectations, and needs. So, how can parents embrace this monumental occasion of bringing a new family member into this world, and still thrive in their personal relationship with one another? Clear communication is the (overly-simplified) answer.

The question remains, however, of "how do I ensure I'm communicating clearly and effectively with my partner?" Luckily you now have access to the answer and it lies in the pages of the book you currently hold in your hands. Kelly Mager has compiled another truly helpful guide to parenting – this time with the focus on Dad! Not only does it contain easy to understand and apply tips and strategies to simplify parenting, it also gives excellent insight on how to communicate effectively to ensure both partners are getting what they need.

When the needs of everyone are understood and met, a truly healthy family dynamic is established, and that is when the happiness and fun begin to shine through!

Terri Di Mauro

The RelationChick

Introduction

Hi dad! You've probably come across this book because someone in your life cares about you, and they know you care about the new life you will be parenting. That person may be a partner or a friend. And maybe this was meant more as a humorous gift – though I hope you'll find it useful as well.

Let's start by talking about the elephant in the room. Why is a woman writing a book about fatherhood? I wrote my first book for moms because I realized how much of the information currently available only talks about funny or entertaining things regarding parenthood. When they happen to mention real problems, they poke fun at them while rarely discussing solutions. Solutions that are dearly needed for one's mental health! A partner's mental and physical well-being makes a world of difference in her ability to handle life as a parent. My first book for mom provides ways to keep her sane.

Upon publishing that first book, the most frequent follow-up question I was asked was "when are you going to write one for dads?" I was surprised by this question because I assumed books geared towards dads would be most relatable coming from a dad. It would have a dad's experiences and vantage point. Wouldn't that make the most sense?

Then I read the books out there...and their reviews.

Although full of personal examples about fatherhood, most read like blog entries with stories detailing their own life. Few provided useful information and tactics that could be applied on your own parenthood journey. Additionally, many of the books only cover pregnancy and birth. Rarely was the nitty-gritty of the first few days, weeks, and years included. Those in the business world call this void a market gap.

As a final call to action, I noticed that many books currently on the market do not fully understand the women's thought process on things. They also contain incorrect or outdated information. This book does not focus on things you are better off reading in a product manual – such as when a child can be forward-facing in a car seat. I'm also not going to cover developmental milestones – stick to a book dedicated to that subject.

What I will walk you through are the easiest and most efficient ways to deal with situations that crop up all the time! Rarely do you read about these subjects. Parents usually only learn about these topics through trial and error. And typically too late in the game for a first child. If siblings join the family later it may get applied, but that assumes you remember!

I don't know why experienced parents don't seem to tell new parents these things – but it's time we did!

I'm coming to you as a mom who developed these skills with my first child. They became even more relevant when 22 months later I also became a mom of twins. Yes, that's right. If you did the math, I had more than a year of telling people I had three kids under age 3!

After writing the initial draft of this book, I made sure plenty of fathers who are past the first year took a look at it. I incorporated suggestions and examples to make this a practical and actually useful handbook for fathers!

This book has been divided into two main sections:

- Things dads wished they knew before having kids so they had a plan in place from the start.
- Things they did to make the act of parenting easier.

So now, dad, let's conquer parenthood. We'll walk through ways to stay sane when it feels like you aren't. We'll discuss common concerns and questions new parents must find answers to. And in the process, you will learn to thrive in your new role!

Part I: What To Know Before Baby Arrives

If baby has already joined your family, read on! This info is still useful and can be implemented starting now.

Knowing about these topics before baby arrives can greatly reduce the stress caused by them. Implementing them after baby arrives allows you to reduce your stress going forward.

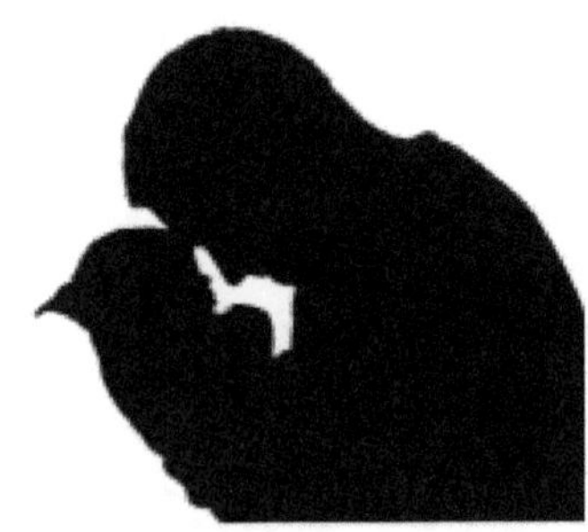

You Are Now An Active Player

O ver the last nine months, you may have gone to doctor's appointments, attended baby showers, and tried to minimize your partner's stress. However, a part of you knows you have little direct control over the baby's growth. Pregnancy and baby's birth is similar to a group class project. One person does most of the work but everyone in the group gets the same grade.

After baby is born, you become a very active player. Your role is important for baby's development and vital to ensure mom is thriving too. Even for a smooth, textbook delivery, giving birth is a big deal. Moms who deliver via C-Sections just had MAJOR surgery.

Why do moms need support just like baby? Imagine completing an Iron Man triathlon. Each day following that Iron Man, you must now complete a sprint length triathlon. You never know when the sprint triathlon will start but must be ready at a moment's notice. That kind of schedule makes recovery harder on mom. It also takes longer.

You may or may not adjust to being a father quickly. Mom may be the same. For all situations, it is important to support your partner as well as the baby as the family dynamic has changed.

Plan for worse than what you expect. Then come up with ideas to handle different situations. This preparation will make you feel more in control when these situations occur. This in turn makes them more manageable.

What am I talking about? Consider what your first weeks with baby and partner might look like if:

- Mom is confined to bed rest for recovery.

- Baby has to spend time in the NICU.
- Breastfeeding isn't going well and you need to feed baby bottles of formula.
- Mom has a c-section or complications that make recovery longer or harder than the average 6 weeks.

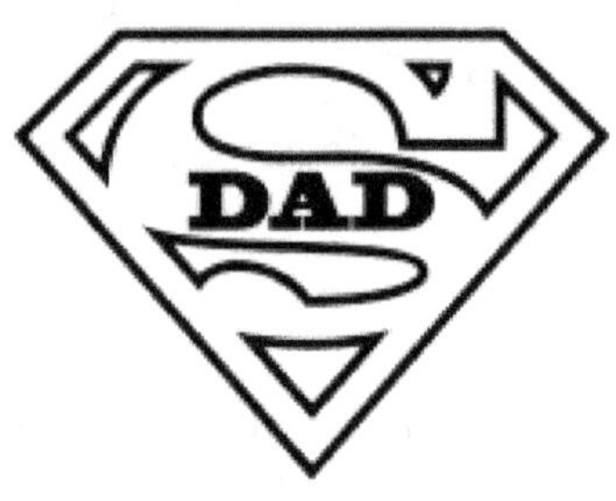

Superdad Tip #1

Actively support both baby AND mom. How you handle and support that transition in the first few months will have a lasting effect on how the next year will go.

Managing Sleep Deprivation

All right, let's talk about sleep deprivation. It's a thing. It's going to happen. There is no way around it. Perhaps you won't take the brunt of it, but that means your partner will. Ever pull an "all-nighter"? Remember how you felt the next day? Now take a variation of that: getting five actual hours of sleep each night. Repeat it night after night, week after week, month after month. And if your situation is anything like ours, it will be years before you get all your sleep hours back. That's going to take a toll on your body and your mental health. It is the same for your partner.

Studies have shown that a week after missing out on needed sleep, your body is unable to recoup the loss, even if you have a chance later to catch up.

There are several ways that you can help minimize the effects that sleep deprivation has on your day-to-day.

Take Turns

One way is to take turns. With a partner in the picture, alternate who is on call each night. This does not create perfect sleep on your nights off. Light sleepers will also get interrupted more. However, you will sleep better knowing you are off duty. In general, you will get more sleep this way and won't rely on the weekend to catch up on sleep.

Team Up

Some couples have great success working together. When baby wakes up, both parents participate. One handles diaper changes and getting baby ready while the other gets set up for feeding.

By doing so, each feeding goes faster. This also means everyone gets to go back to sleep sooner.

Week Vs Weekend

Another option is having one person in charge at night (typically the woman, especially if she is breastfeeding). In exchange for being in charge during the night, she gets more breaks during the day. This can include sleeping in on your days off and taking naps. This is the arrangement my husband and I use to this day. It allows him decent sleep on work nights, and I get a few extra hours each morning when he doesn't need to go into the office.

Trade Nap Times

During the day, you can take turns with who is on duty with baby and who can relax. This is easiest to implement if you are home with baby due to paternity leave, your work schedule, or other circumstances. You can nap when baby naps, or just as easily when your partner is feeding or playing with baby. After your nap, swap responsibilities. Repeat as necessary.

I highly recommend having a discussion with your partner about each person's expectations for getting enough sleep. Get enough sleep so you can function well and keep family harmony. One of you may require more hours than the other to feel that way.

As a note, c-sections, multiples, and complications may temporarily change your agreed upon system. With a c-section, it can be hard and painful for her to get out of bed by herself, or bending down to pick up or put baby in bed. With tandem feeding multiples early on, it is hard to properly support their heads and bodies while getting both into position to eat at the same time without help.

Furthermore, I'll point out here that most mothers wish for more sleep as a Mother's Day Gift. We'll take that over flowers, fancy dinners, and cute personalized gifts any day when our sleep tank still needs recharging.

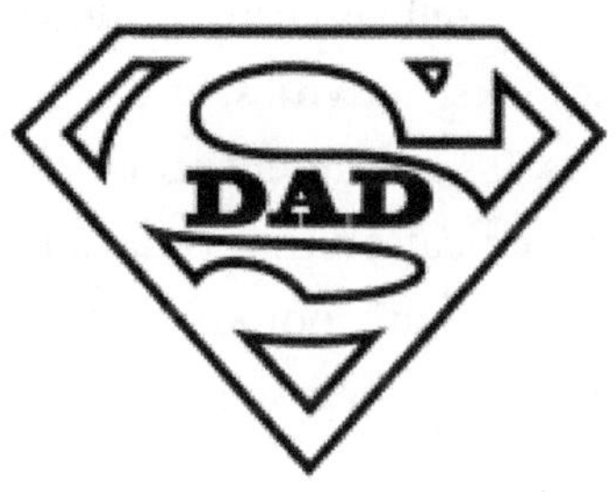

Superdad Tip #2

Create a system to ensure you and your partner get enough sleep throughout the week.

Me Time/Hobbies

Before kids, time to yourself was usually dictated by your preferences. You chose your hobbies, activities, and work schedule based on all of your needs. After kids, it's a different story. Your time now requires a new level of scheduling dedication that is hard to picture until you have to do it. Let's be honest, your bathroom time is no longer your own when a little one always wants you in their sights!

You are still a person with needs and wants of your own. It is important that you continue to nurture things that have meaning for you. It also helps to create time daily where you can get a break from parenting and work. The same goes for your partner. Make sure you spend this time doing something you truly enjoy. Doing so should re-energize you.

The best way to ensure you have some "me time" for you, and your partner gets theirs as well, is by scheduling it. Babies are notorious for working on only their schedule, so you have to ensure someone else is watching baby for this period of time.

It's also important in these early months while exercising your "me time" to assign timelines and adhere to them for your partner's sanity. This predictability makes it easier for either of you to handle a child or children by yourself, knowing that your partner will be back at a certain time to take over or co-parent. Make sure you honor these time commitments. Leave at the planned time and return at the planned time.

Let's throw in a personal example. Shortly after our twins were born, my husband was invited to join a friend for a river kayak trip. He had not done the route before and was told it would take 2 - 2.5 hours. Add in the time it takes to reach the location, unstrap the kayak, etc, and I knew this excursion would be at least 3 hours worth of time. I agreed to it. 3

hours passed with no sign of his return. There were no calls or texts with an update. I started to feel a rollercoaster of emotions. Annoyed because that is a long stretch of time to yourself on a weekend with three young kids at home. Frustrated because I had no update on when I might expect him, and anxious because I also became concerned that something had gone wrong. I was stressed. Turns out the friend who invited him had not kayaked that route before and had estimated how long it would take to complete. My husband had not wanted to contact me until he knew where they were and when they might be able to exit the river and return. His total time gone was 6 hours. Afterward, we discussed the need for more accurate info, and adhering to the agreed timeline we give the other when enjoying our "me time".

Make sure that you choose activities for your "me time" that refill and recharge you mentally and physically. Do not feel you have to use it for certain things because that's what others do. Choose the activities that make you feel like yourself afterward. Moms are big culprits of saying "me time" is going to the grocery store without kids. For the record, it's not. There may be a few people out there who love shopping so much that the grocery store counts for them. For most, think more along the lines of:

- Video games.
- Golf.
- Reading.
- Exercising (at a gym or in nature like hiking/biking/kayaking).
- Attending a sporting event.
- Working on cars/motorcycles.
- Bar night with the guys.

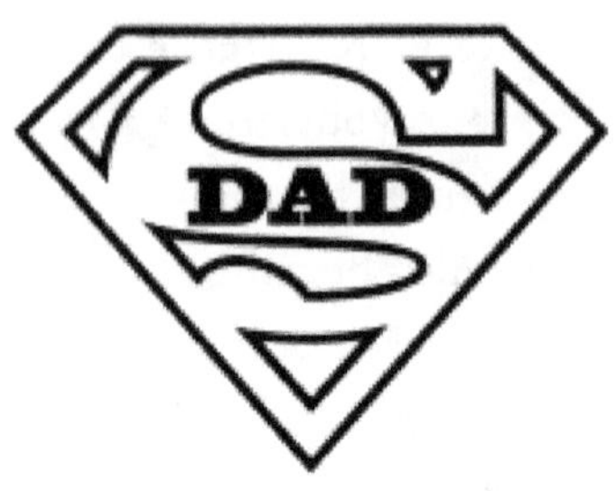

Superdad Tip #3

Schedule time daily to focus on you and recharge.

Household Chores

This is a category that can morph drastically over time. You have probably already experienced this with a variety of roommates, whether it was at college, living alone, or after getting married. The key here is to communicate and come up with a distribution of chores that is agreeable to both of you.

Let's elaborate. Before baby, chores were probably organized based on each person's skill level and time available to complete. These were then referenced against each person's preference for doing one thing over another.

For instance, my husband doesn't like grocery shopping and I do it since I don't mind. After the baby, I continued to do so because my husband would rather have the kids by himself for a full day when I go than spend 2 hours grocery shopping each week.

On the other hand, if I did the cooking we would be eating scrambled eggs, smoothies, and other things that do not require turning on the oven. We also would not have a single spice in our pantry. My husband enjoys cooking and promptly added 20 spices to our pantry when he took over. He also uses the oven frequently.

We care so much about each area that no matter how cranky the kids are during the time these items need to get done, we'd still rather watch the kids than trade.

Some changes to chore responsibility may be temporary based on your child's age, a switch in living situations, physical ability based on health, or available family and friends that can help.

You may have this discussion with your partner and end up agreeing you can both carry on as before. This may be built on ideas such as "I can do laundry while baby sleeps", not knowing that baby will want to nap on someone every day for a period of time.

Perhaps you think some items can be accomplished while baby is in a wrap or carrier, only to find out your child hates it.

You may decide to set aside money so you can pay someone to take care of some items. Plan for both a one time job, or regular sessions for a season of your life.

When discussing your plan, consider how frequently a chore needs to be done. That first summer after having triplets the lawn might not get mowed as often. Fall chores that used to take one weekend to complete might get spread over a month. Open and honest communication on how much you care about certain items will help you both reach an agreement.

It's good to come up with a plan, but successful implementation means checking in at regular intervals to assess if it is working. Be flexible and step up when needed if life isn't going as planned. A partner will do the same for you. Any choices you make can be revised again as your baby and family dynamics change. What is important is seeing and responding to them.

Want to supercharge your superdad powers? Without being asked, take care of something falling through the cracks. These efforts really are appreciated and recognized even if they forgot to tell you.

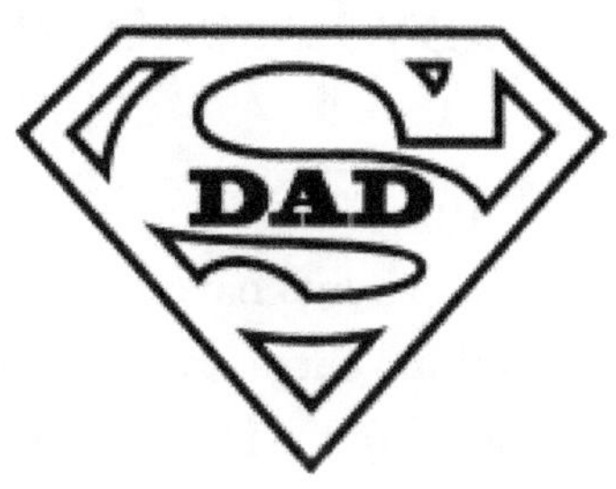

Superdad Tip #4

Come to an agreement on chore responsibility and touch base
occasionally so things don't slip through the cracks.

Basic Baby Essentials, Etc

It seems all books for new parents have a discussion point over must have items and what to skip. There are probably more blog posts on this topic than I care to think about. My book for moms includes a list of things I recommend borrowing rather than buying. I am including some of that info here as a starting point of reference.

The list of things you can buy for your child(ren) never ends. Products are added daily to stores hoping you will buy them. This is especially true if you absorb a lot of media. I liken this stage to being engaged and evaluating wedding options. Between The Knot, Pinterest, and pictures on any wedding photographer's website, you learn that options for your wedding are endless. The bare requirements include a courthouse ceremony and marriage certificate. Everything else is extra. Extras may change the vibe, make the wedding day easier on the couple, or end up not getting used. However, each item you add costs money or time.

With that, you can consider things for children in the same way. The bare essentials are a safe place to sleep, some clothes, diapers, food, and the most important thing – love! After that you can make choices on items that will make your life easier, keeping in mind not every baby likes every baby device on the market.

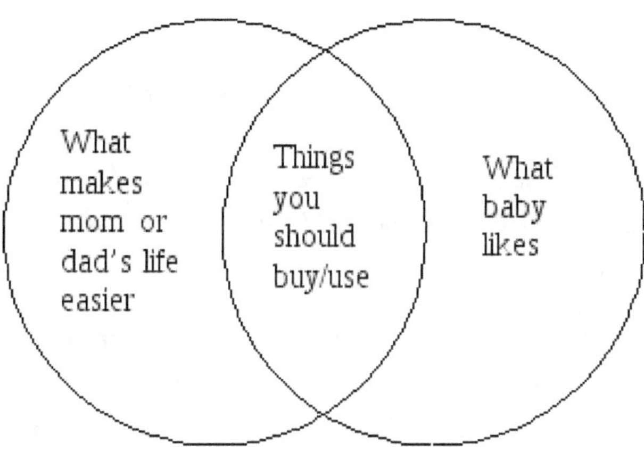

One great way to find the center of a Venn diagram between "what makes mom's life easier" (dads too as this info also helps you!) *and "what baby likes" is to borrow. Ask families with older children to borrow an item during its limited use time frame and return it when baby outgrows it.*

Or, borrow long enough to know if your baby likes it before purchasing it yourself. Many moms keep things for later down the road and are happy for it to get additional use in the meantime. This arrangement also frees up their storage space for a bit. Pay it forward by being one of these moms when an item is not in use.

Consider borrowing the following items:

- *Bassinets.*
- *Swaddles.*
- *Baby bathtub.*
- *Bouncers.*
- *Exersaucers.*
- *Types of baby carriers (soft, hard, front carry, back carry, wraps, slings, etc).*
- *Swings.*

- *Playmats.*

We borrowed a swing when the twins arrived. Although we used it on occasion, I was so glad we didn't spend the money on our own. I would not have felt the purchase price justified the use it got. By borrowing, we had it when we really needed it and were able to return it without guilt after the boys outgrew it.

After borrowing an item, if it falls into your Venn diagram circle, make the purchase. You'll know it was the right one to help you out, relieve your stress, and make baby happy. This will also minimize instances you may be at your wit's end and shop online for a solution. No one likes having buyer's regret when Amazon delivers the purchase the following day, only to learn baby hates it.

If you don't have people you can borrow from to test items out, consider online marketplaces and buying them used.

Below I will touch on baby basics most people consider. Thinking outside the box can save you time, money, and allow you to re-purpose them after your child has outgrown the original intent.

Swaddles

Most babies love to be swaddled, even if they don't act like it. They were tightly confined in the womb, so that sensation is comforting to them. To swaddle a baby, you can use a blanket, sleep sacks with velcro that are faster and easier to use, and products like the Magic Sleep Suit. Receiving blankets are best used when baby is not sleeping.

Bed

Baby can only sleep in one place at a time. That said, in my opinion, the only thing you need to have is a Pack 'N Play with a bassinet level option.

Perfect for anyone without a lot of space, on a budget, or if you plan to move the location where baby sleeps over time.

The baby industry will try to sell you on a variety of cribs or bassinets. Here are the additional reasons I recommend only having a Pack 'N Play:

- You only have to purchase one item. This saves money and space.
- It can easily be moved upstairs or downstairs and between rooms in a house. This is helpful if mom struggles with the stairs in the early days after birth, as well as if baby starts in your room and later moves to another.
- It packs down small for travel. This makes them great for trips to visit family/friends and for vacations. It provides a familiar place for naps in a new location.
- Most have a bassinet level that reduces how far you have to bend down until baby weighs 15 pounds (check manufacturer instructions for other considerations on limits).
- Cheaper than most cribs.
- Babies won't be chewing on wood or ingesting paint while teething – it's very common for kids to gnaw on the top railings later on.
- Baby's arms and legs won't get stuck sticking out between the bars (Pack n Plays have small mesh netting).
- Pacifiers and other items are less likely to fall out due to the netting mentioned in the bullet point above.
- They are made to be quick to assemble.
- They are readily available second hand at garage sales and consignment sales – this means you can buy one cheaply and can easily resell after it's no longer needed.

White Noise Machine

I highly recommend something to create white noise in baby's room once baby becomes more alert. This does not have to be an actual white noise machine. A small portable fan will work just as well and can be easily repurposed after it's no longer needed for white noise.

Phone apps to create white noise also exist. Make use of an old bluetooth speaker or phone/tablet to be your white noise machine.

Diaper Changes

Every time I see a post or read an article that talks about a parent's irritation at getting peed or pooped on, I am surprised. As a caregiver, you will be intimately involved with your child's bowel movements while changing diapers and potty training. Fact: you will get peed on. Fact: you will get poop on you. Just not necessarily when or how you might expect.

One way to simplify this process is to keep all diaper changing items ready at hand in a designated location. This can be in a diaper bag, a basket, a spare bathroom, or other places that works well in your home. Diapers will get changed in a lot of weird places. However, having a consistent place you keep supplies will help.

Do you want to avoid being peed on in the middle of diaper changes or during bath time? Then any time you perform a diaper change, offer baby the potty. Especially for boys, the cool air when a diaper is removed prompts them to pee if their bladder is full. Do the same thing when undressing baby for bath time. Have him sit on the potty to pee while you run the water.

When baby is small, they will need your support for this process. Act as a chair by holding them under the thighs with baby's back against your chest. Andrea Olson of GoDiaperFree.com has a wide variety of resources to help with this. Understand that your child knows more than you think when it comes to bodily functions!

Bath Time

Many people make bath time a routine part of getting ready for bed. First, if bath time is not a calming activity for your baby, it does not need to be a daily part of the bedtime routine. Secondly, baby does not need to be cleaned daily. They may get messy from pee or poop, but you are cleaning that up during diaper changes. It is perfectly acceptable to go several days between baths. None of my kids liked baths early on and we only bathed them one time per week. It saved our sanity as adults and resulted in less crying for them.

Pajamas/Clothing

Here is another area where I would say pick your battles. Pjs can be comfy. However, if your baby or toddler would rather not have a wardrobe change going into bedtime, choose if you want this to be part of your routine. As long as our kids' clothes are relatively clean and appropriate for the nighttime temperature of the house, we let them sleep in their daytime clothes. We decided early on there were other parenting items we cared about more. Changing our stance on this made bedtime shorter and less stressful for everyone.

This applies to clothing in general. Let them dress themselves. Let them go without. Summertime, potty training, and illness are all times where clothing and type of clothing is subjective.

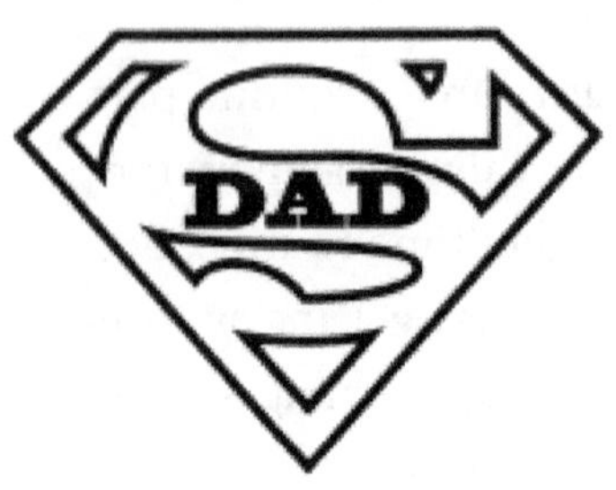

Superdad Tip #5

Save space, money, and time by borrowing items, re-purposing others, and only purchasing once you know it benefits baby AND you.

Connecting w/Partner

Gary Chapman wrote a book called "The Five Love Languages". His book discusses how people value things and actions differently than others. He then walks you through questions to help determine your primary love language as well as your partners (you can take the test at https://www.5lovelanguages.com/quizzes/). Learning your primary love languages helps you understand what your partner appreciates, and why it may be different than your own.

For anyone unfamiliar with the five love languages, I have listed them below.

- Words Of Affirmation.
- Quality Time.
- Physical Touch.
- Acts Of Service.
- Receiving Gifts.

I wrote the first draft for this section on Mother's Day. This may surprise some of you. It comes down to my love language preferences that my husband understands. My primary language is 'acts of service'. By allowing me to sleep in, work on a project of my own, and have some quiet time while he manages the kids, he is showing that he understands me. He is giving me the type of love I most value and appreciate.

In contrast, 'receiving gifts' ranks last for me. Therefore, expensive gifts including flowers or dinner out mean little to me.

Why am I talking about a book someone else wrote? For starters, once you become a parent, understanding what your partner values is more important than ever. Your free time and mental bandwidth are mostly consumed by your children. You want every action you take to maintain and cultivate your relationship to count. Rather than using all five methods evenly, make sure to identify and use the one(s) your partner values most. Think of it as getting the most bang for your buck.

There is another important reason I bring up these five love languages. Once you transition from a couple to a family with a child, they will evolve. In general, I'm not talking about the rankings changing, though they could. It is the way each love language can be met and expressed.

Here are examples for each.

Words of Affirmation

As a couple: I love spending Sunday brunch with you.

As a family: I love watching you play with the kids.

Quality Time

As a couple: Checking out a local event you both enjoy.

As a family: Netflix and chill once the kids are asleep.

Physical Touch

As a couple: Anything that could count as a public display of affection.

As a family: Getting lots of cuddles and bonding moments with baby.

Acts of Service

As a couple: Holding doors open or mowing the lawn.

As a family: Feeding baby, taking care of the car oil change, planning vacations, washing the laundry.

Receiving Gifts

As a couple: Flowers and other sentimental gifts.

As a family: Massage gift certificate or night off from performing bedtime routines.

Notice how you can still fulfill your partner's primary love language after baby is added into the mix. It looks different in my examples and may vary further with your partner. Not sure how to adjust? Go ahead and ask. It may sound like "I know how much you loved xx before baby arrived. I know that doesn't fit easily into our life anymore. Is there something I can do instead?"

I have one more thing for you to consider. Your baby also needs to receive these love languages. Their preferences will shift more in the early years based on their needs and development. Sometimes you can help the most by providing a love language to your child that your partner struggles to give themselves.

This can be cuddling your child if your partner gets touched out more quickly, taking on more of the diaper changes, and letting baby hear your words of affirmation.

PS – if your partner gets touched out during the day from all the physical contact with their child, consider that impact on your relationship with them. What would happen if you take on some of that load?

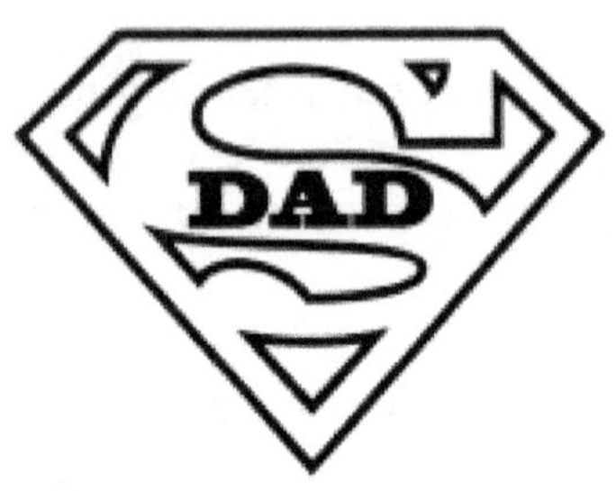

Superdad Tip #6

Utilize your partner's primary love language often. Understand that how you express it may look different now.

You Can Handle It On Your Own, But You Don't Need To

We spent the first few years without any close family nearby. With 3 kids under age 3, we didn't want to impose. Our kids were a handful by themselves. So we mostly did it on our own. You don't have to. Take advantage of offers and help you receive from friends and family.

Utilizing this network is good for your children and extended family. Your children will get experiences they may not have with you and allows your extended family to build closer bonds with your children. Everybody wins!

Friends and family will not offer to do something they are actually unwilling to do! These small breaks can provide needed time to recharge your energy. Just as taking some time for yourself gives you a mental break, mini breaks offered by family and friends are also beneficial.

When our kids got a little older and my parents were visiting more often, we would snatch two hours on a weekend morning to take our road bicycles out together. It was wonderful to get some fresh air and exercise as a couple.

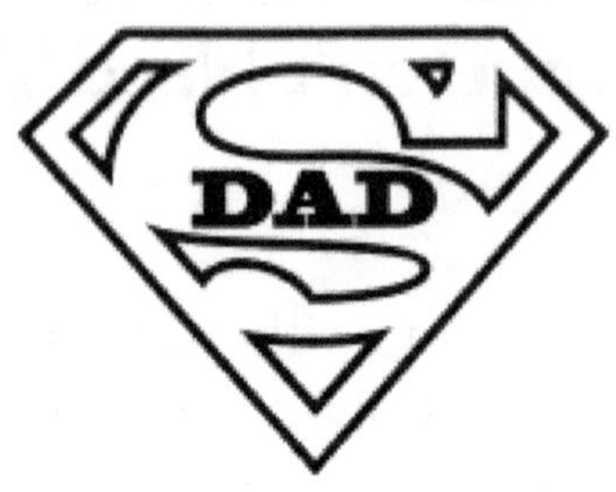

Superdad Tip #7

Take friends and family up on their offers for help.

Learn To Prioritize

This book focuses on things you can do to be a superdad. Part of being a superdad is understanding your limits and prioritizing help items that will be most effective. No one can do it all every day. You will need to figure out what is important and prioritize it.

This is something you may have found a rhythm for at work. Make sure you do the same at home. With whatever schedule you come up with, remember it'll require a certain amount of flexibility, as well as being manageable and maintainable for the long haul. Things to consider:

- Exercise.
- Family time.
- Housework.
- Time with friends.
- Continuing education commitments.
- Me time for both you and your partner.

My husband and I utilized the weekend downtime when the kids were sleeping for priorities that were otherwise hard to do.

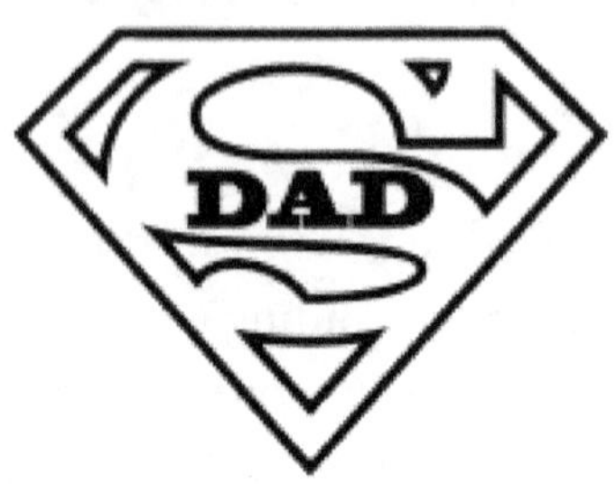

Superdad Tip #8

Identify and schedule your day based on the importance of each activity. Create a system that can withstand the long haul.

Part II: How To Make Parenting Easier

Parenting is a hard job. Unlike previous generations, we have access to information they never did. It is easier than ever for people around the world to share ideas and knowledge on any topic, including this book. This section discusses effective actions you can take to make parenting easier. Learn from the moms and dads that have gone before you!

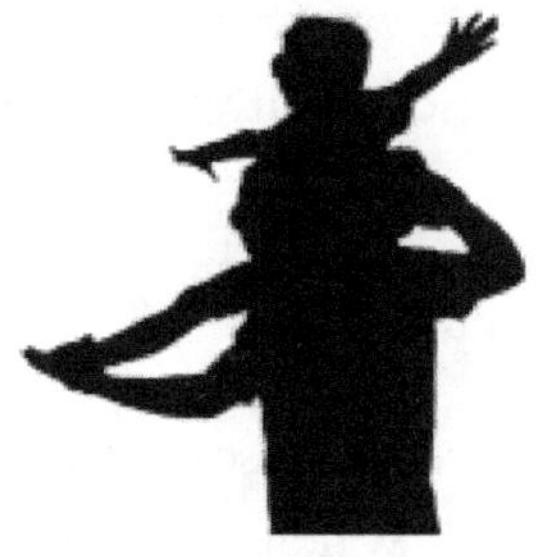

Kids And Physical Space

In a few other sections, I mention how much children like to be around you. It bears repeating. They want to be around you. All. The. Time. In the bathroom. When you're showering. If you're cooking or cleaning. While you talk on the phone. When you get the mail. As you wash the car. The list goes on.

There are a few different reasons for this. First, they love you. They love being near people they trust and love. It makes them feel safe and secure. Second, they love learning. Things we've done for most of our lives and consider mundane are brand new to them. They want to see what you are doing, why you are doing it, and how it works. They want to know if they can participate.

When possible, engage that curiosity.

Keep this in mind as you recreate personal space and borders. This will shift as your child ages as well. When your child wants to help and you invite them to participate, <u>consider the importance of the journey</u>, and not just the destination. When you do so it will be a good experience for you both.

What types of journeys am I thinking of?

Chores

Cooking, and other household chores. Have them around, and eventually helping with weeding, picking up sticks, taking out the trash, and more. It may take longer this way, but you are also bonding with your child. You will have more success here by giving them direct, specific tasks to do. Consider phrases like "please put these cups away", and "will you get a washcloth for me?"

Play

Playtime, including reading. There is no "right way" when it comes to exploring books, blocks, sand, water, music, and more. The act of play itself is better than having a perfectly designed fort last through the play session.

Activities

Including items as simple as walks. Yes, you might be walking around the neighborhood and be focused on a nonstop trip. You may be used to this early on when baby is sleeping in a stroller and you dictate the speed and length of the walk. However, unless you have a strict time limit before the next activity, stop to look at bugs, talk with friends, and discuss what causes the wind to blow. I once had a 1 mile walk with my oldest when he was a toddler that took an hour. At times it pained me to stop so soon after we had begun moving again, but his fascination and interest during the walk made me rediscover the scenic view around me.

You can choose the level of involvement for activities where age, skill, and understanding play an important part. They may not be able to do everything in a given activity. But involving them where they can allows you both to learn and bond together.

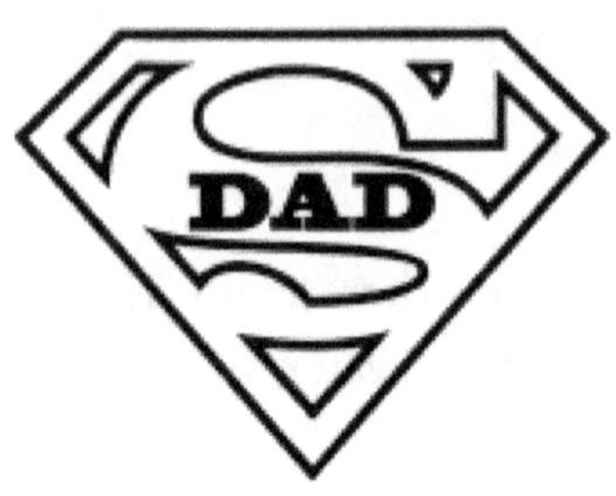

Superdad Tip #9

View your child's experiences and curiosity from their perspective and form thoughtful boundaries you can both respect.

Go Outside!

This may feel like an obvious thing. Of course you'll spend time outside!

Have you heard of seasonal depression? There are links between sunshine, vitamin D, and people's moods. When there is a lack of sunshine, many feel less happy. Now apply that to children who are not able to regulate their emotions and feelings, nor able to communicate them. Spending time outside provides a wealth of benefits. Reference the outdoor education program Tinkergarten[1] for a better understanding of how playing and experiencing nature helps children. As a parent, time outside aids in re-calibrating sleep cycles for nap time and night time as well as calming them.

If you aren't already familiar with the "witching hour" and colic, you probably will be soon. These typically occur during the time after your child's last nap and before bedtime. They are cranky because they are tired, but not so tired as to fall asleep for the night.

Many times when my husband and I were not sure what else to try, one of us would take the child in question and step outside our front door. Doing so was like flipping a switch. Their inconsolable crankiness was immediately replaced by a calm and quiet baby.

Water is also a part of nature. Whether you engage with it outside or in the bathtub, your child may be equally calmed by playing with it. Make sure to have a few scoops and buckets available to enhance the experience. Measuring cups work great!

---

1. https://tinkergarten.com/

Nature soothes and engages their minds without being overstimulating. Use this to your advantage.

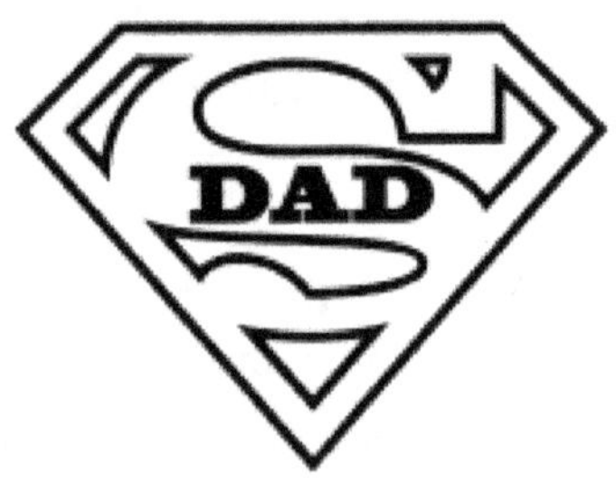

Superdad Tip #10

Utilize outside time and water play to calm even the crankiest child.

Looping In Your Partner

After a vacation, most people need time to decompress from it and get looped in on what has happened while they were gone. This can be at work and home. Usually both.

In a similar vein, you will want to do the same thing regarding baby. Whoever has left baby gets a few minutes to transition to being at home. Then, offer to watch the kid(s) for a bit. This gives your partner a break and allows them to mentally offload. It might be used to make notes on something, use the bathroom in peace, or spend time clearing their head. Doing so will make the next hours easier.

Use this time to ask questions and exchange information. Knowing about diaper changes or bathroom breaks are just as helpful as how much time was spent outside, how many books were read, and how long baby may have napped. These updates can help prepare you or your partner for what the next several hours will likely look like.

If one of you works outside the house all day, it may be helpful to provide an occasional text update, email, or phone call to prepare the other for a certain situation.

For example, the first time my twins skipped their only nap of the day, I was frazzled from not getting a break. I was tired from trying to get them to nap unsuccessfully. And I knew that meant they would go down for bed early that night.

A heads up to my partner in this situation is nice because he already knew I was tired, was prepared for cranky kids, and understood dinner needed to be cooked as soon as he got home so everyone would have a chance to eat dinner before bed.

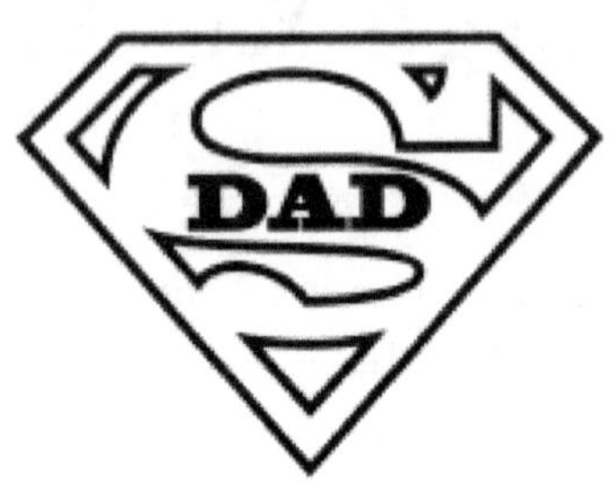

Superdad Tip #11

Check in on how things are going with your partner and return the favor so each has an idea of how the day went and what to expect next.

Read

An easy activity that benefits kids is reading. Library cards are your friend and well worth it for the variety of resources and activities they have. Many libraries go beyond books, carrying puzzles, games, audio books, music, magazines, newspapers, and toys. Libraries also maintain online educational subscriptions including courses and languages. Some offer less obvious choices including telescopes, sewing machines, cake pans, or metal detectors that you can explore with your child. Many items are available in both physical and digital forms.

As a bonus, reading benefits your child at every age.

Newborn babies love to hear your voice. Reading provides an easy way to talk to your baby. While snuggling into you and listening to your voice, they will be content to listen for about as long as you are willing to read.

From six to about eighteen months, books are an interesting tool for motor skill development. I rarely read past page two on a book before they were ready to get the next one. However, turning pages, looking at and talking about pictures, and sharing touchy-feely stories make for great fun. They became acquainted with the idea books can be lots of things.

Around eighteen to twenty-four months, your child will want to listen to books again. Kids thrive on repetition and will pick up new things each time from the stories. It helps them learn to anticipate actions, grasp a story's flow, and get a feel for sentence structure.

Reading time is a great way to bond with and continue to strengthen your relationship with your child. Even if you are not an avid reader yourself, I bet you will enjoy and be entertained regarding things in each stage of your child's development and their enjoyment of books.

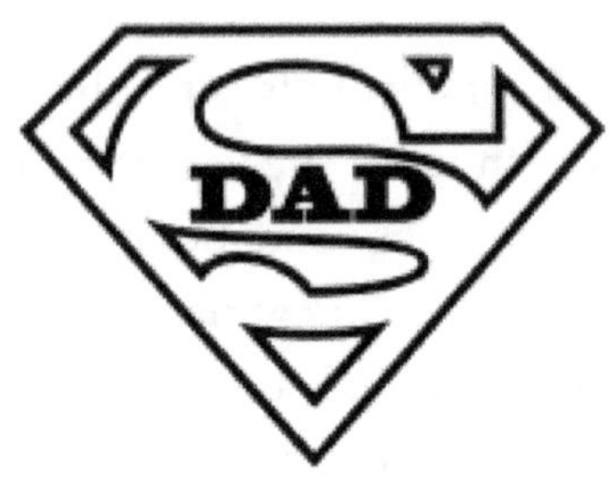

Superdad Tip #12

Reading books is a great go-to idea for interacting with your child at every age.

You Are Enough

As a parent, our natural desire is to fix things for our children. Early on, those things are basic. You help with diaper changes, feedings, snuggles, and sleep.

As your child ages, other skills will be developed. During the learning process, there will be many instances where they get upset while trying to accomplish something new. For many children, the simple act of being there for a hug or a kiss when they need you is enough. They will cheerfully bounce off for more fun and another try. Do not assume you need to fix things. Giving them a safe space and your support is typically enough to bolster their resolve before jumping into the next thing. Check out the children's book "The Rabbit Listened" by Cori Doerrfeld if you doubt this concept.

Following this thought process, ensure they get opportunities to grow without stepping in and doing it yourself. As mentioned earlier, let them enjoy the journey, not just its completion. Kids develop at their own rate. Respect their wishes, and make sure they know you are available if they want assistance.

The concept of You Are Enough covers a wide range of activities. Immediate standouts from our parenting journey so far include:

- Feeding self.
- Learning to walk.
- Learning to dress themselves.
- Any sort of play where they are being challenged with new skills or concepts (building towers, using tools, cooking, etc).
- Getting hurt during an activity they were having fun with.

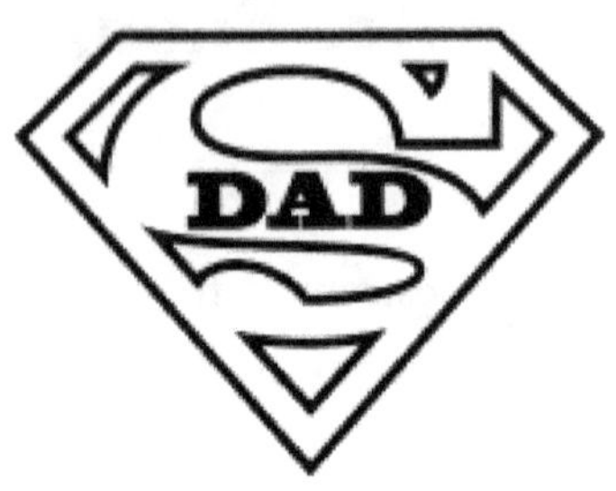

Superdad Tip #13

Kids view parents as their safety net. They are more confident to learn and try when they know they have your support. Being there is support enough in most instances.

Set Expectations

Your child will not be purposely deciding what happens each day. They will, however, end up dictating some of what happens as you accommodate their sleeping, eating, and awake times.

You and your baby will find a rhythm that works for your family. Be protective of that schedule when setting expectations for your day. Many parents find that consistency in sleep times eases the process of going down for a nap or at night time.

And just as you enjoy knowing what to expect for the day, so will your child. So go ahead and loop them in. You don't have to give the itinerary for the whole day early on. Start with your current activity and what comes next. Doing so will make transitioning easier. If you don't, expect a fuss if your child is engrossed in something.

This is something you already do for yourself. When you aren't in charge of the schedule, it becomes more important. Think about a time things were going well. You were enjoying yourself. Then you get a phone call saying it's time to come home and get ready for an event. An activity you had not been told about before you left.

Do you feel frustrated? I'd answer yes. Few people like to be pulled out of an enjoyable activity. Some of the enjoyment from that activity has probably evaporated too. Not to mention that the next one may not sound like fun or something you want to get to on time.

Let's compare it with this next version. You agree with your partner that you will be leaving for some "me time". There is an agreed on amount of time because immediately afterward the family is leaving for an event.

In the latter version, when it is time to break away from your "me time", you probably didn't feel the same emotions. Perhaps a reluctance to return home, but knowing full well you got the time you asked for and knew the time given was in relation to leaving for the next activity.

Your child will appreciate the same types of notice for transition times. Of course a newborn can't tell time and won't be able to visibly react and acknowledge a time routine early on. However, just as you can generally tell what time of day it is before checking your clock, your child can also get a sense of time and understand when you give it a label.

Providing activity change warnings will make breaking from one activity to the next less jarring for everyone. Having a loose routine for each day gives children structure and a rhythm to follow. They won't get caught off guard when it is time to change activities, even ones that have their full attention.

Here are some conversation examples about timing and routines:

- We have 10 more minutes of story time, and then we are eating lunch.
- After breakfast we are going outside for a walk.
- Our car ride today to get to the park will take as long as it takes to get to the library.
- Inside the library we will return books, attend story time, then come home for a nap.
- You may have a snack after being buckled into your car seat.
- Mom is making a stop at the bank drive-thru on the way to the park.
- We are going to Max's house for a play date. We are staying outside the whole time.
- It's 5 minutes before bedtime. It's time to clean up the toys.

If those sound overwhelming, a general "5 more minutes!" before switching tasks or changing locations works well.

Furthermore, it's no secret that it will take you longer to do something or go somewhere with baby. It will only stress you out more if that timeline is gets pushed to the limit from a poop right after strapping baby into the car seat, almost forgetting an item you have to take with you, or the flustered feeling you get after wrestling with baby regarding clothing, shoes, or car seat straps.

Manage your expectations by building a buffer into all these activities. Everything takes longer with kids. You may end up somewhere early. You may have to leave an event before it's over to make your next engagement (even if that engagement is normal bedtime). And you may get little else done except a core goal set for the day. The good news is that creating a buffer is a lot less stressful than rushing. Plan an extra 10-15 minutes into any activity, transition time, or other commitment to minimize the stress you get from toeing the line too close. This includes days you don't even leave the house!

Bedtime and nap time warnings have been a consistent help for my boys and me. When you do create a bedtime routine, I suggest you build in a countdown notification. We started our routine when the children were around six months old. I give them a warning 10 minutes before we go upstairs to brush teeth, potty/diaper, and read a story. This way they know the night is winding down, but that they still have time to finish their current activity/play. Other ways to facilitate the bedtime transition include lowering the lighting and avoiding rambunctious activities.

We give another warning at five minutes which signals the start of toy cleanup. All toys must be put back in the toy bin in some fashion. Originally mom and dad did most of the work. Now that our youngest are toddlers, our children are responsible for completing the task. When cleanup takes more than five minutes they know that this means they will lose some reading time.

After cleanup is done, we say it's bedtime and head upstairs for that process.

This routine initially resulted in some whining, and it occasionally crops up again. Most days, however, the boys are excited and ready to go upstairs. They race to be the first one to get their toothbrush, though not necessarily to get their teeth brushed. I owe their cooperation to the routines and expectations we established early in their lives.

Additionally, at the end of a long day, there is something satisfying as a parent in giving those countdowns. You know the end is near and how much time is left to hold it together before decompressing afterward.

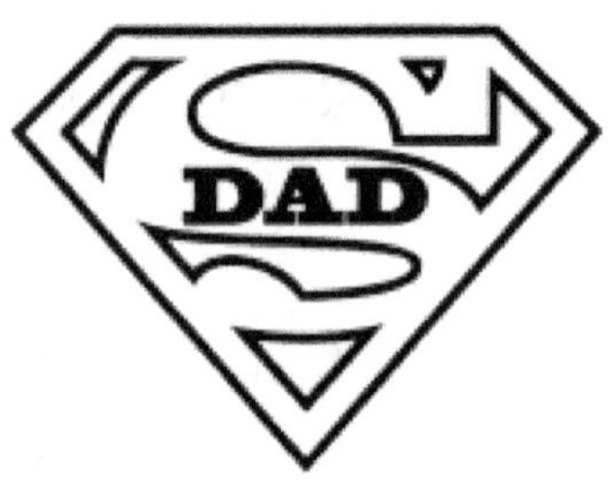

Superdad Tip #14

Set expectations for yourself and your child to help with transition times.

Bright By Text And Imagination Library

These two free services -Bright By Text[1] and Imagination Library[2]- provide an easy way to stay abreast of your child's developmental milestones. Sent to you at regular intervals, they also contain ways to interact and encourage your child in their learning.

BrightByText.org is a nationwide program available in English as well as Spanish. After providing your phone number and age(s) of children in your family, they will periodically send you age development information and resources to support your child with those milestones. If your local county also participates, you can learn about free, local events and activities to attend.

During pregnancy, some parents do a lot of reading about raising a baby until they become a moving toddler. Once you are busy raising baby, finding time to read, let alone choose which books to read, becomes harder. By this time parents typically only dive back into parenting books after a problem crops up. Bright By Text allows you to be a little more proactive in your role as a parent without spending a lot of time on it.

Dolly Parton's Imagination Library sends you a book each month that is geared toward your child's age until they turn five years old. These books cover a wide range of topics. Each also includes suggestions for questions you can ask and ways you can use the book to teach various concepts. Learn more about the program as well as its availability where you live at https://imaginationlibrary.com/.

---

1. https://brightbytext.org/

2. https://imaginationlibrary.com/

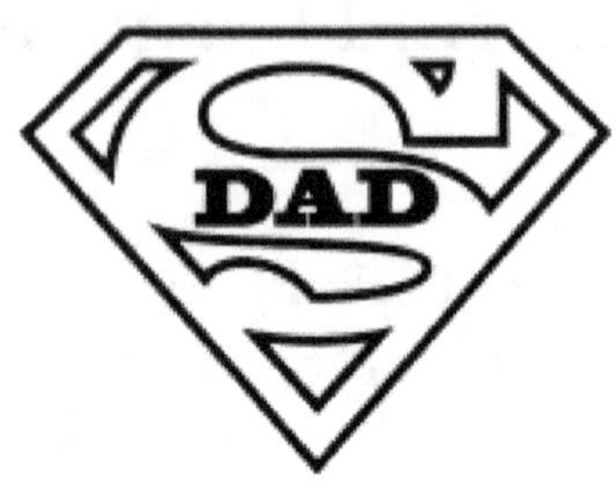

Superdad Tip #15

Utilize resources for prompts on learning and activity ideas.

Handle Your Own Family

Some amount of time after getting married, I came across the idea that if I was upset about something my partner did, I would be better off discussing it with my partner's parents rather than mine.

The concept is that my partner's parents would still love and forgive him. The in-laws may even provide insight from the years before I met him regarding the issue in question.

On the other hand, talking with my parents would inevitably tarnish their view of him. And they may wonder if my partner was good enough for me.

Now add grandchildren into the mix. Having boundaries and situations addressed by the blood-related parent imply that both you and your partner agree on them. A grandmother is more likely to listen to their own child rather than the in-law about their grandchildren's boundaries and rules.

Take this mental load off your partner's head. Handle inquiries, questions, and any drama that arises from your side of the family. You may need to consult your partner on opinions and stances before responding to your family.

If this idea makes you uncomfortable, I encourage you to check your feelings if the roles were reversed. This applies to small and large communications alike.

Common items we each address with our respective parents and extended family include gift ideas, parenting decisions around how we are raising our children, and travel plans.

You know your side of the family best. This means you may need to be the primary communicator regarding other situations or in different ways. The same goes for your partner.

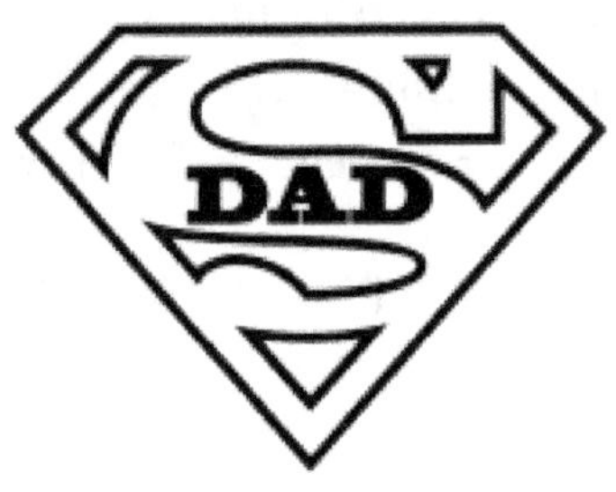

Superdad Tip #16

Take the lead on any communication needed with your side of the family.

Understand Your Area Of Influence

As a parent, part of your job is to set expectations and guide the course of the day for you and your child. Some of those expectations will be on how you want to parent and how you would like your children to behave.

You will, however, need to let go of any ideas you have about being in absolute control. No matter how much you would like to think of your child as an extension of yourself or your partner, they are their own person. This becomes more apparent the older they get. And that person wants to learn, test, and experiment in ways you cannot imagine now.

This is where understanding your area of influence becomes helpful. You are not able to force your child to sleep at a certain time. You can, however, place them in a dark room at a comfortable temperature with a self-soothing object and remove all distractions.

Sometimes that will work, and other times it won't. When you try to control all aspects of a situation, the job of parenting becomes overwhelming and more stressful. This is an easy way to lose any enjoyment it would have brought.

This area of influence can crop up in any situation. A child who wants to skip a nap or is dropping a nap is a prime example. Don't forget the fun idea you have for a game that your child chooses to play differently. These situations may zap your excitement away. Think how they feel if the roles are reversed.

Instead, try creating the rules and play parameters together and see what happens! Luckily, this can go both ways and I am constantly amazed at my kid's imagination for activities I worried they wouldn't like. Are you teaching them to blow bubbles in the water? Stick your fingers underneath and ask them to "blow out the candles"! Are you hoping they'll help you weed the garden? Challenge them to find the next weeds for you to get and ask if they are strong enough to carry tools around to help you.

Kids love showing you what they can do. Many times all it takes is asking. Use that to your advantage.

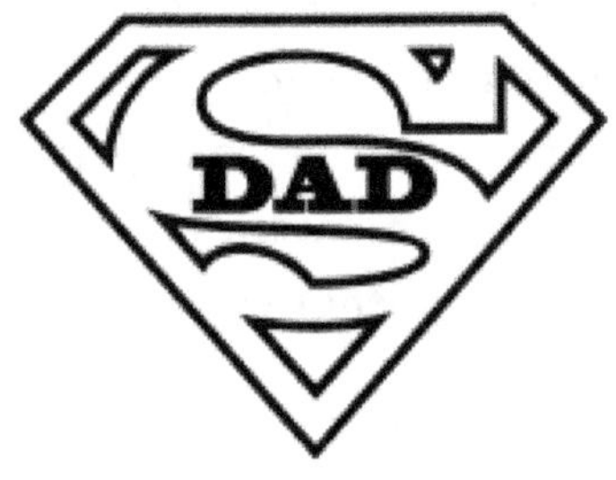

Superdad Tip #17

While you cannot make your child do everything, utilizing play and staging the setting can help you achieve the desired outcome.

Conclusion

<hr>

You've probably noticed that most of the ideas presented in this book are interrelated. Kids are curious, experimental, and ambitious in their mission to learn about the world which surrounds them. These tips should help you manage the early years with fewer surprises and a quicker learning curve.

Remember that families are to love and enjoy. Find things to do together. Families are not meant to make us look good or stress us out. Although I hope they bring you joy, it is not a child's responsibility to make you happy. Nor is it your job to make sure they are always happy. Giving in to their every demand may make them happy now, but creates a bad habit and poor coping skills when they become an adult.

You are now equipped with some of the most helpful tips and tricks that experienced parents wish they had learned sooner. I can't wait for you to be a superdad in your own family!

<hr>

Want to help others decide if this book is right for them? Leave a review!

The Superdad Superspeedy Tip Recap

———

All of this books tips located in one spot for fast access!

Superdad Tip #1

Actively support both baby AND mom. How you handle and support that transition in the first few months will have a lasting effect on how the next year will go.

Superdad Tip #2

Create a system to ensure you and your partner get enough sleep throughout the week.

Superdad Tip #3

Schedule time daily to focus on you and recharge.

Superdad Tip #4

Come to an agreement on chore responsibility and touch base occasionally so things don't slip through the cracks.

Superdad Tip #5

Save space, money, and time by borrowing items, repurposing others, and only purchasing once you know it benefits baby AND you.

Superdad Tip #6

Utilize your partner's primary love language often. Understand that how you express it may look different now.

Superdad Tip #7

Take friends and family up on their offers for help.

Superdad Tip #8

Identify and schedule your day based on the importance of each activity. Create a system that can withstand the long haul.

Superdad Tip #9

View your child's experiences and curiosity from their perspective and form thoughtful boundaries you can both respect.

Superdad Tip #10

Utilize outside time and water play to calm even the crankiest child.

Superdad Tip #11

Check in on how things are going with your partner and return the favor so each has an idea of how the day went and what to expect next.

Superdad Tip #12

Reading books is a great go-to idea for interacting with your child at every age.

Superdad Tip #13

Kids view parents as their safety net. They are more confident to learn and try when they know they have your support. Being there as support is enough in most instances.

Superdad Tip #14

Set expectations for yourself and your child to help with transition times.

Superdad Tip #15

Utilize resources for prompts on learning and activity ideas.

Superdad Tip #16

Take the lead on any communication needed with your side of the family.

Superdad Tip #17

While you cannot make your child do everything, utilizing play and staging the setting can help you achieve the desired outcome.

Did you love *New Job: Dad*? Then you should read *15 Ways For New Moms To Manage Stress And Stay Sane: The Actually Useful New Mom Care Package*[1] by Kelly Mager!

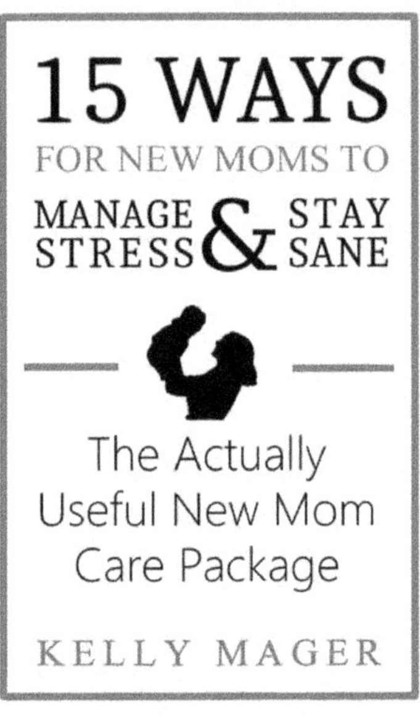

[2]

The perfect baby shower or new mother gift!

Written by a mom who had three kids under age three for over a year. Edited and influenced by moms who are past the first year. Made for moms who want to:

Learn about ways to organize their day and manage their expectations.Discover how to tap into their local community, family, and friends for support.Minimize stress caused by four main money concerns by implementing provided strategies.Maximize their mommy/baby bond with four parenting frameworks.

---

1. https://books2read.com/u/31YOxW

2. https://books2read.com/u/31YOxW

As a new mom, ease your transition into motherhood with 15 ways not commonly written about that moms use to manage their day to day.

Get a handle on your stress levels, stay sane, and find new ways to enjoy the everyday in every day, starting today!

Read more at https://amzn.to/3kJVOFH.

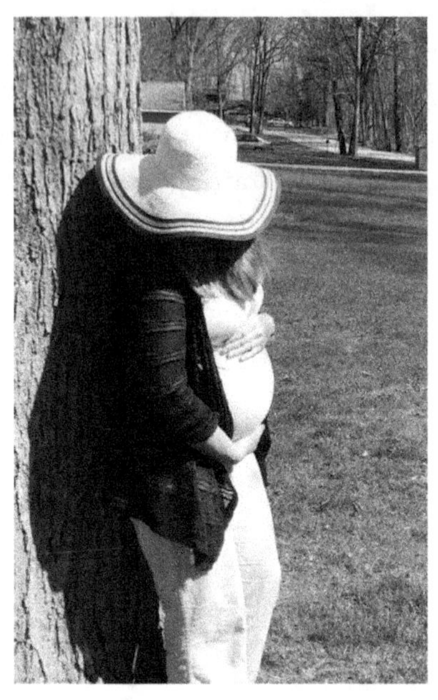

About the Author

Kelly enjoys most articles that depict aspects of raising children. However, she has often been disappointed in products advertised as helpful to new moms since they have rarely been helpful to her. This inspired her to connect parents with meaningful resources to make life easier, more organized, and better supported. She kicked off her mission with the publication of "15 Ways For New Moms To Manage Stress & Stay Sane: The Actually Useful New Mom Care Package". Learn more about her current projects on Instagram, Facebook, and Etsy at MiniMischiefManaged.

Read more at https://amzn.to/3kJVOFH.